Table of Contents

COPYRIGHT

Introduction

The menopause means the last menstrual period but many women will talk about 'going through change of life. when discussing the time from when they first notice changes in their monthly cycle and the start of symptoms such as hot flushes up to and after having their final period

Every woman will go through the menopause and for each the experience will be different. The menopause doesn't begin at a particular age or last for a definite and fixed period of time and the symptoms can vary from woman to woman.

For some the menopause can pass with no problems but for many others the time can be very unsettling and for some women the menopause and its symptoms can be so difficult to manage, particularly in the workplace, that they make the decision to give up their employment rather than continue to struggle in an environment that is unsupportive or lacking understanding of their needs at this point in their lives.

What is the Menopause?

The three stages of menopause:

> ➢ Peri-menopause – the stage from the beginning of menopausal symptoms to the post-menopause

> ➢ Menopause – the last menstrual period

> ➢ Post-menopause – the time following the last period, usually defined as more than 12 months with no periods in someone who has their ovaries or immediately following surgery if the ovaries are removed.

The menopausal period is the point in a woman's life when her periods become more irregular and infrequent and then eventually stop.

For many women the menopause occurs as they age and the ovaries naturally fail and stop producing the hormones oestrogen and progesterone; for others the ovaries fail due to specific treatments such as chemotherapy or radiotherapy or when the ovaries are removed, often at the time of a hysterectomy.

The average age for a woman to reach the menopause is 51 but a woman can start to experience natural menopausal symptoms between the ages of 45 and 55.

The peri-menopause is the time when a woman's periods become less frequent until they stop altogether, for most women the peri-menopause can last for several years (the average is four but it can last for up to ten years), however for a few women periods may stop suddenly rather than decreasing over time – for these latter women symptoms can be worse. During peri-menopause the reducing levels of the hormone oestrogen can cause physical and emotional symptoms such as hot flushes, night sweats, mood swings and vaginal dryness.

The menopause is the last period/bleeding. Women are said to have reached the menopause when they haven't had a period for 12 months.

Post menopause is any time after the last period.

A diagnosis of a natural menopause is made from a combination of factors with most emphasis being placed on the pattern of periods and the presence of menopausal symptoms. In the late 40s and early 50s the absence of periods or infrequent periods along with symptoms such as hot flushes can alone be used to diagnose the menopause and blood or urine tests are unnecessary. In women under 50 the menopause is diagnosed after 24 months without a period, for women over 50 the menopause is diagnosed after 12 months without a period.

Early and Premature Menopause

Before the age of 45 the menopause is referred to as early menopause and a menopause that starts before the age of 40 is called premature menopause. Both early and premature menopause may also be referred to as premature ovarian failure and about 1% of women under 40 and 5% of women under 45 will be affected.

In many cases there is no cause but premature ovarian failure can be caused by such things as:

- Hysterectomy

- Certain types of radiotherapy and chemotherapy

- In rare case some infections such as TB, mumps, malaria, varicella (the virus that causes chickenpox and shingles) and shigella (a type of bacteria that causes dysentery)

> Certain medical conditions such as enzyme deficiencies, Down's Syndrome, Turner Syndrome, Addison's Disease and hypothyroidism (under-active thyroid)

Women affected should see their GP for possible referral to a gynaecologist as treatment may be needed to ease menopausal symptoms and prevent osteoporosis; they will also be able to discuss fertility issues (a small number of women who experience premature menopause may still have intermittent ovarian functions so they may still be able to conceive).

Symptoms

It is thought that changing hormone levels cause menopausal symptoms in about three quarters of women, with lifestyle factors such as diet and exercise and certain medications also influencing women's experience in the run up to menopause.

The first symptom is usually a change in the monthly period with light or heavy periods and irregularity in their occurrence (you may have a period every two or three weeks or you may not have one for several months). Other symptoms can include physical, psychological and sexual problems such as:

- ➢ Hot flushes
- ➢ Night sweats
- ➢ Insomnia
- ➢ Palpitations (heartbeats that suddenly become more noticeable)
- ➢ Headaches
- ➢ Aching joints, muscles and tendons
- ➢ Irritability and mood swings

- ➢ Anxiety and panic attacks

- ➢ Poor concentration

- ➢ Poor memory

- ➢ Loss of sex drive

- ➢ Discomfort during intercourse (caused by vaginal dryness)

Later symptoms due to lack of oestrogen can affect the bladder and vagina and can include needing to urinate more frequently and discomfort when doing so, increasing urinary tract infections, bladder leakage and vaginal discomfort such as dryness, burning and itching. The skin can become dryer, thinner and more prone to bruising and hair may thin and dry. Unwanted facial hair growth can also be explained by lack of oestrogen.

Other symptoms experienced during the menopausal period by some women are:

- ➢ Itchy skin, sometimes with the feeling that something is crawling on them

- ➢ Light headedness/dizziness

- ➢ Tingling in the arms and legs

- Burning sensation in the mouth

- Tinnitus

- Breast tenderness (and they may shrink slightly!)

- Fatigue

- Gastrointestinal upset such as indigestion, diarrhoea, wind and bloating

- Increase in allergies

- Change in body odour

- Bleeding gums

- Changes in the fingernails

- Feelings of unspecified fear and dread

As can be seen from the wide range of symptoms it can be difficult to recognise what it is happening as a part of the menopause and many women don't realise that they have entered the peri-menopause as they continue to have periods. Any symptoms should be noted and a doctor's advice sought if they are severe or are impacting on your quality of life.

The severity of symptoms and the overall duration of the menopause vary, depending on factors such as lifestyle, genetics, stress and overall health.

Managing Your Symptoms

Many women are able to manage the symptoms of the menopause themselves, simple diet and lifestyle changes and easy self-help approaches can help to relieve symptoms and these are discussed below.

For those with more severe symptoms or symptoms that interfere with their day-to-day life there are medications available. The type of treatment will depend on the individual and professional medical advice from your doctor should always be sought in these case

Diet

During the menopause falling levels of oestrogen will reduce the amount of calcium in your bones; women who aren't using Hormone Replacement Therapy (HRT) are particularly at risk from this. Decreasing bone density can lead to osteoporosis, see below. In addition during the menopause a woman's risk of heart disease increases, see below, and weight gain can become more of an issue (reduced muscle mass can mean less calories are needed daily).

A healthy, balanced diet should provide a good supply of calcium, tips for healthy eating before, during and after the menopause include:

> Eat less saturated fat

> Choose lean cuts of meat

> Choose low or reduced fat dairy foods

> Reduce salt

> Eat at least 2 portions of oily fish a week

> Eat at least 5 portions of fruit and vegetables a day

> Include plenty of fibre in your diet

Exercise

As well as having a healthy diet regular exercise is an important part of staying healthy during and after the menopause. There is some evidence that women who exercise regularly and are more active tend to suffer less with menopausal symptoms.

In addition to the benefits of exercise on the symptoms of menopause there is the additional benefit of protecting the body from osteoporosis and heart disease. Exercise helps to keep muscle and bone strong, increasing flexibility and mobility and improving balance.

The best exercises are those that are aerobic, sustained and regular, for example running, cycling and swimming along with strength and flexibility exercises. For women who have never taken regular exercise or haven't exercised in a long time brisk walking three times a week is a cheap, easy and good way to start exercising if you previously haven't been active.

Always talk to your doctor before taking up a new exercise programme particularly if you have osteoporosis or other health conditions or concerns.

Alcohol

Cutting down on your alcohol consumption at any time can have a positive effect on your health and this is also true for women during and after the menopause.

There is anecdotal evidence to suggest that for many women alcohol consumption increases during the menopausal period. This can be for differing reasons, for example some may see drink as a way of getting to sleep when they are experiencing insomnia; others may see it as a way of coping with stress or forgetting their problems for a time.

In addition to the symptoms of the menopause there are many other changes that may be potentially impacting on a woman's at that stage of their lives – children growing up, parents growing old, bereavement, marital changes, divorce, all can have an effect on emotional wellbeing and drinking to overcome these emotional difficulties or indeed increased opportunities for social drinking can all lead to increased alcohol consumption.

Alcohol however can increase the severity of the symptoms of menopause and can be a trigger for hot flushes and night sweats. Though a drink before bed may help sleep what is experienced isn't a restorative sleep.

Alcohol is also a depressant, though initially there may be a feeling that the stresses and worries of the day have been lost through a glass of something nice, ultimately heavy drinking can contribute to feelings of depression and anxiety and can make coping with stress more difficult.

Drinking more than recommended guidelines can increase the risk of breast cancer in all women, and the risk can increase further in women using HRT.

Women who smoke have an earlier menopause than non-smokers, have worse hot flushes and often don't respond well to tablet forms of HRT.

Hot Flushes and Night Sweats

This is the most common menopausal symptom and each hot flush in general lasts for 4 – 5 minutes.

> ➢ A hot flush is a sudden feeling of heat in the upper body; it can start in the face, neck or chest before spreading upwards and downwards.

> ➢ The skin can become patchy and red and you may start to sweat.

> ➢ The heart rate can also change becoming very rapid or irregular and stronger than normal (palpitations).

> ➢ Hot flushes that happen at night are called night sweats.

> ➢ Most hot flushes will only last a few minutes.

> Hot flushes can occur before your period stops but are most common in the first year after the final period and last on average for two years; for about 10% they can continue for more than fifteen years.

Although the exact cause is not known, falling levels of oestrogen would seem to have an effect on the body's temperature controls. Body temperature naturally goes through a pattern of rises and falls through a 24 hour period which usually goes unnoticed; during the menopause the changes caused in the temperature control area of the brain mean that women may flush with a temperature rise, even moving from a cool room to a warm one or having a hot drink can trigger a temperature rise that leads to a hot flush.

For many women the effect of hot flushes in work can be a problem to manage - being unable to cool down through opening a window or using a fan and wearing uniforms made of man-made fibres for example. In addition the potential for embarrassment when in highly visible tasks such as meetings and events can be very distressing for many women.

It can be difficult to completely stop hot flushes and night sweats but their intensity and frequency can often be reduced. Using a combination of the following approaches can help:

- ➤ Wear natural fabrics such as cotton and dress in layers that can be easily removed when needed.

- ➤ Use cotton sheets and layers of bedding.

- ➤ Open a window or use a fan to keep the room cool at home and at work.

- ➤ Have cold drinks in preference to hot drinks.

- ➤ Try to lose weight if you are overweight or obese.

- ➤ Eat a healthy diet

- ➤ Take more regular exercise.

- ➤ Try complementary therapies such as yoga or controlled breathing;

Keep a record of when you have hot flushes to try and identify what triggers them, this may be getting too warm, drinking hot drinks or alcohol or eating spicy food. If your record helps you identify a pattern in your flushes you may be able to avoid the trigger and reduce the frequency and impact of your flushes. Even without identifying obvious triggers a record can help you measure the impact of other approaches you are using.

There are also medications, including hormone replacement treatment (HRT), that your doctor can prescribe to help reduce the intensity and frequency of your hot flushes.

Insomnia

Night sweats and anxiety can lead to many menopausal women suffering insomnia, this in its turn can lead to irritability and problems with concentrating and forgetfulness.

Along with the advice above for hot flushes and night sweats the following can help you to relax and sleep well:

- Avoid exercising late in the day (within 2 hours of bedtime).

- Have a warm, not hot, drink, brush your teeth and maybe read in bed – a regular habit such as this can let your brain know that it is time to sleep.

- Go to the bed at the same time and get up at the same time every day – too much time in bed can affect quality of sleep leading to tiredness in the day.

> If you can't sleep get out of bed and try reading or listening to some quiet music. Go back to bed when you feel tired.

> Breathing exercises and relaxations techniques can help reduce stress and sleeplessness.

If insomnia is a problem and the above approaches don't help your doctor may be able to prescribe medication for a short time that could help in re-establishing your sleep pattern. Or try Hyponis there are so many free setions on You Tube and they help, a lot.

Frequently Urinating

During the menopause you may need to pass urine more often, have some leakage or be more prone to urinary tract infections.

Try to drink plenty each day, at least 2 – 3 pints (1.5 litres) to keep your bladder healthy – not drinking enough can cause urine to become concentrated and this can then irritate the bladder potentially leading to urinary tract infections. See your doctor if you suspect you have a urinary tract infection – symptoms include cloudy or smelly urine and a burning sensation, discomfort or pain when passing urine.

Doing regular pelvic floor exercises (Kegel exercises) can help strengthen the muscles that hold urine in the bladder and prevent leakage.

Skin Problems

Skin problems during the menopause are linked to hormonal changes in the body. Women may experience dry skin; oily skin; itchy skin (pruritis); pins and needles or tingling or pricking sensations (paresthesia) and for some a sensation described as like having insects crawling over the skin (formication).

Oestrogen stimulates the production of collagen and oils through oestrogen receptors in the skin. Therefore as oestrogen production slows during the menopause the skin often becomes dry and itchy, though this is more common in the years immediately following menopause for some women the changes begin in the peri-menopause.

Self-help for skin problems during the menopause include:

> diet – eating healthy fats such as salmon, walnuts and eggs

> applying sunscreen even on an overcast day

➢ avoiding piping hot showers and baths - choose warm water instead

➢ drinking plenty of water

➢ using gentle soaps

➢ exfoliating regularly and applying moisturiser daily

➢ reducing alcohol consumption

➢ giving up smoking

Itching and other symptoms may be caused by the lowering oestrogen levels affecting the receptors in the skin. For itching symptoms, over the counter antihistamine creams may help or if symptoms of itching, pins and needles, tingling or skin crawling are impacting on day-to-day life advice can be sought from your doctor on medical treatments such as HRT.

Menstrual Changes

Many peri-menopausal women find that their menstrual cycle and flow changes. Some women may experience irregular periods that stop and start with no apparent pattern. It is also common for women to get heavier, lighter or longer periods at this time. Some women also report that the colour and texture of the blood appears to change with some describing the consistency as 'globular'.

The erratic nature and unpredictability of periods during this time can be embarrassing and sometimes debilitating for women, never knowing when a period will start and whether the flow will be heavy means that it helps to be organised, carrying sanitary protection at all times.

It should be noted that irregular or heavy bleeding can sometimes be a symptom of other problems, including polyps, fibroids and cancer, so women experiencing this should always consult their doctor to ensure that heavy or irregular periods are menopause related. A doctor can also provide advice on treatments such as HRT and the coil to manage and regulate menstrual bleeding and can test iron levels to ensure heavy periods are not causing anaemia.

It is important that any bleeding 12 months or more after the last period is investigated by a doctor.

Vaginal Dryness

Lowering levels of oestrogen can cause vaginal dryness and itching and can make sex uncomfortable or painful. About a third of women will experience this during the perimenopause and it becomes even more common after the menopause.

Medical advice should be sought from your doctor who can provide guidance on treatments available. Treatments that you use should be reviewed regularly and you should inform your doctor of any new symptoms you may have.

Some of the treatment creams available can damage diaphragms and condoms so you may need to use another form of contraception to avoid pregnancy.

Vaginal symptoms are likely to continue or worsen without treatment.

Lower Sex Drive

This is a symptom of the menopause that can also be affected by hot flushes and vaginal dryness. Treating these two symptoms can help to improve your sex life but where a problem persists HRT is usually the most effective treatment. HRT isn't recommended for all women, particularly those who've had breast cancer. Seek advice from your doctor on treatments and other support available.

Psychological and emotional symptoms such as depression, anxiety, poor concentration, mood swings, irritability, forgetfulness and sadness are all common during the menopausal period.

Hormonal changes can be attributed to some of these symptoms, but the other changes in a woman's life at this time should also be considered in relation to their impact on mental wellbeing.

The menopause can occur at a time of other major changes in life – the death of parents or aging parents who may be becoming more dependent; children leaving home; divorce or the death of a partner and physical aging. Other challenges can include beliefs about no longer being useful, a fear of death, a distorted body image and feelings of low self-worth.

It is for these latter reasons that it can be hard to tell whether psychological and emotional symptoms are directly related to the menopause - studies have shown however, that women who are generally happy in their lives experience fewer problems during the menopause.

The psychological effect of physical symptoms is important too. For many women a hot flush may be a relatively minor inconvenience that will pass in time, but for others the distress, shame and negative thoughts that they engender around being out of control, being embarrassed and a feeling of aging may mean that they resent the symptoms and suffer psychological distress as a result.

The important thing to realise when considering the psychological and emotional symptoms of the menopause is that they are real. There can be a tendency to dismiss mental health problems and, when the reasons for the problems can be unclear and complex, choice of treatment may not be easy and will vary according to the individual.

There are different treatments available for psychological and emotional symptoms, some will require intervention and referral from a medical professional such as your doctor, and others are self-help techniques that may help improve mood and emotional wellbeing. By following the approaches above to manage hot flushes, night sweats and insomnia, taking regular exercise and trying different relaxation techniques such as yoga and tai chi you may be able to improve your mood.

Medical Treatment for Your Symptoms

Many women don't need treatment for the menopause as symptoms are mild and can be managed without medication. However medication may be recommended when symptoms are more severe and impact on day-to-day life.

Treatment options include:

> Hormone Replacement Therapy (HRT)

> Tibolone (similar to HRT)

> Clondine

> Vaginal lubricants

> Anti-depressants

Menopause, Pregnancy and Contraception

Although pregnancy is less likely around the menopause, over the age of 40 it is still important to use contraception if you wish to avoid unplanned pregnancy.

During the peri-menopause a woman's periods may become irregular and unpredictable but her ovaries are still likely to be producing some eggs, so though natural fertility does decline pregnancy can happen.

To avoid an unplanned pregnancy some form of contraception is recommended until the menopause – the NHS recommends using contraception until 2 years after the last period or bleeding if under 50 years of age and 1 year if over 50 years of age.

The choice of contraception when over 40 can be influenced by a number of factors:

> How effective the method is

> Possible risks and side effects

> Your natural decline in fertility

> Personal preference

> Other medical conditions that should be considered

Several forms of contraception will need to be prescribed by your doctor after discussing the above factors. Natural family planning is not recommended for peri-menopausal women as a form of contraception as irregular periods can make predicting ovulation difficult.

It is worth noting that the combined oral contraceptive pill can mask the symptoms of the menopause (such as hot flushes and night sweats) and withdrawal bleeding will continue while the pill is being taken so it is hard to know if you are still fertile or indeed if you are post-menopause – speak to your doctor for advice on determining if you are postmenopause if you are over 50 and using the pill as contraception. Doctors may prescribe the pill to some women to help with menopausal symptoms such as hot flushes and irregular and heavy periods.

HRT is not a form of contraception and will not stop you becoming pregnant.

Risks for Menopausal Women

Osteoporosis

An important effect of reducing oestrogen levels is an increased risk of loss of bone strength leading to bone thinning (osteoporosis). Women are more at risk of developing osteoporosis then men because of the hormone changes that occur during the menopause – oestrogen is essential for healthy bones and when its levels fall bone density is directly affected.

Women are at greater of risk of developing osteoporosis if they have an early or premature menopause, if they have a hysterectomy where the ovaries are removed before the age of 45 or if they have absent periods due to over exercising or dieting.

You can reduce the risk of developing osteoporosis by:

> Doing short, frequent sessions of weight bearing exercise

> Eating calcium rich foods

> Quitting smoking

> Moderating your alcohol consumption

Heart Disease

As oestrogen levels fall its protective effect on the heart is lost and changes occur that can lead to an increased risk of heart disease. Women are three times more likely to die of heart disease as of breast cancer and in the years following the menopause the risk increases significantly. The changes and risk factors include:

- Obesity – more common in women than men over 45 years of age. During the menopause the body fat distribution changes from the 'pear' shape to the' apple' shape

- Cholesterol – menopause is associated with a gradual increase in cholesterol and particularly bad cholesterol

- Hypertension/High Blood Pressure

- Smoking

- Diabetes

- Low levels of exercise

- Alcohol

Menopause Myths

The menopause begins at 50. The menopause is the last menstrual period. As mentioned earlier the average age for the menopause is 51 – 52 but the menopause can happen before or after this age. Women may experience perimenopausal symptoms before they have their last period. These symptoms may start a few months, or up to 13 years in some cases, before menopause

You will gain weight during the menopause. The lowering levels of oestrogen can lead to reduced muscle mass meaning that the body no longer needs as many daily calories as previously. As stated earlier by following a healthy diet and taking regular exercise weight gain can be prevented. Where you may notice a difference is in the distribution of body fat, with more being stored around the stomach rather than on the hips and thighs.

There's no difference between surgical and natural menopause. Surgical and natural menopauses are very different. When a woman undergoes a total hysterectomy she will experience an immediate and significant change in hormonal balance rather than the usual more gradual change in natural menopause.

The first sign of the menopause is a hot flush. Symptoms in the perimenopause are varied and a hot flush may not be the first sign that your body is entering this stage of your life. Tiredness, anxiety, irritability, mood swings, depression, weight gain, hair loss, cravings, poor concentration, forgetfulness, irregular periods, heavy or light periods and lowered sex drive can all be symptoms of the peri-menopause. With so many different possibilities many women don't recognise their symptoms as being due to the start of their peri-menopause.

After the menopause you no longer produce hormones. During the menopause oestrogen and progesterone levels do decrease but they continue to be produced, just in smaller amounts post-menopause

The older you are on when you start your period the older you will be when you go through the menopause. For many women the opposite is true!

Predicting the age of your menopause is very difficult but there are some questions to think about:

> What was your mother's age at menopause, the age she began to experience symptoms can be a good indicator for you too

➢ Do you smoke as this can cause earlier menopause

➢ Do you drink daily as drinking alcohol can mean a later menopause?

➢ Have you been pregnant, more pregnancies suggest later menopause

Menopause only causes physical symptoms. As can be seen above the

menopause doesn't only cause physical symptoms. Many women experience

psychological symptoms such as anxiety, depression, forgetfulness and poor memory.

Some of these symptoms can be exacerbated by physical symptoms such as night sweats

and hot flushes.

The best way to get through the menopause is HRT. For many women selfhelp approaches are enough to allow them to confidently manage the symptoms of the menopause. For some women other health considerations (such as premature menopause) or symptoms that seriously impact on day-to-day living may mean that HRT is needed.

Being aware of your options is important in ensuring your mental and physical wellbeing during and after the menopause. Talk to your doctor about your symptoms and choices.

Advice to Other Women

Don't expect to have problems. No all women have problems through the menopause; many women have either no symptoms or intermittent symptoms which have little impact on their lives.

Talk to people, get support. There are some women who feel very isolated through the menopause, maybe feeling embarrassed to discuss their symptoms. Rather than keeping quiet and trying to cope alone it's important to talk to people – friends, family, partners and colleagues. Sharing your experience and speaking out can mean you find support and discover many others are going through similar things. See the information at the end for details of national support groups.

Be informed. Every woman's experience of the menopause is individual and unique, knowing about the changes your body is going through, talking to people, reading and searching for information on the internet can better help you understand what is happening. Some women on Healthtalk.org felt that doing their own research on the internet helped them find the information and support that hadn't been provided through their GP – which had been very clinically focused.

Seek help. Sometimes managing the menopause alone becomes impossible and knowing when to seek medical advice and developing a good relationship with their health professionals was important both during and after the menopause. Women on Healthtalk.org suggest contacting your GP if you have heavy bleeding or emotional problems and also keeping a really detailed diary of symptoms so that a GP can be in a better position to give advice.

Be assertive. The importance of being proactive and assertive in managing the menopause is stressed. Taking charge by asking questions, keeping asking until you get helpful answers, doing your own research so you are sure what you are asking and changing GP if necessary are all given as suggestions for keeping control when menopausal symptoms are making life difficult.

Consider a range of treatment options. Finding the right treatment for you can be difficult, what works for one woman may not work for another. For some women HRT is the solution for others its simple lifestyle changes such as diet and exercise.

Women who had used HRT successfully to manage their symptoms stress the importance of finding out as much as possible about risks and benefits before making a decision.

Keep healthy. Paying attention to diet, exercise and lifestyle can help women through the menopause. Many women have stressed the importance of eating well and exercising in how it made them feel.

Keep the menopause in perspective. As well as keeping healthy, women stressed the value of maintaining a positive state of mind. Whilst acknowledging that the menopause can be a tough time for some women their message was not to let it take over your life or use it as an excuse to stop doing what you want to do.

It's important to remember that though for some women the menopause may be a time of regrets (feeling older, passing child bearing years) for many others it is a positive time, a new chapter, with opportunities to discover new interests and friendships, to try new things, to get fit and healthy and to learn new things about themselves.

There is also advice on the same site for partners of women going through the menopause – the understanding and support of your partner is important at a time when symptoms both physical and psychological can place a strain on your relationship.

Foods For Menopause

What is it about the change of life that has a woman scrambling to find the right food for menopause? Besides the loathsome middle age spread, besides the fact that her body is betraying her by wanting her to slow down, a woman at menopause will be seeking better food for menopause to regain her health. Or she should be, at least.

The metabolism slows down because the body wants to hoard all the resources it can. It has sensed that a major change is going on, which puts stress on the body. Stress triggers adrenalin and cortisol, the "fight or flight" hormones, and, instead of helping the woman, she finds herself depressed, and likely seeing the beginnings of some very serious disease processes.

So, good food for menopause will help a woman, in numerous ways, to regain her health posture and remain vital and active. What constitutes good food for menopause?

Wholesome food tops the list, and that means the menopausal woman needs to eliminate the bad foods from her diet. Bad foods include refined sugar, highly processed foods and white flour products, as well as excessive caffeine.

Eating foods as fresh as possible and that are processed with less chemical processes are best. A diet rich in protein, low in fat and balanced for vitamins and minerals, makes the grade for the food for menopause diet.

Vegetables and fruits contain all the necessary vitamins and minerals a body needs, but supplements can be added in, especially in areas where certain foods are just not as readily available. For example, areas where fish is not a major food source will find people lacking in fatty acids like Omega3, a very necessary ingredient for good health. If fish is not favourable to you for your food for menopause diet, then adding an Omega3 supplement is recommended. The same goes for other necessary foods items, like soy and calcium.

Red meat should not be on your list of food for menopause, although it can be consumed in moderate amounts. What you want is lean meats that are very high in protein.

Water is life, as they say, and drinking plenty of water is important. If you liken your body to a car and your food for menopause as the fuel, then water is like the oil in the car. It keeps the systems cooled and lubricated.

One way to tell if you are dehydrated is to notice how often you get constipated. When the body is dehydrated, the bowels are the first place the body goes for the fluids it needs. So, literally, everything flows much more smoothly when there is plenty of water available.

Foods to Avoid

In general, the typical Western diet of white flour, and full-fat dairy and meat is not only unhealthy but also contributes to hot flashes.

Avoid chemicals that mimic estrogens (xenoestrogens) found in pesticides or herbicides by eating organic foods.

Intensively reared animals have often been treated with antibiotics and hormones, another reason to eat organic meat and chicken.

Minimize your exposure to foods stored in plastic containers and never heat or microwave food in plastic containers - as they will leach xenoestrogens.

Cut down on all caffeine, fizzy cola-type drinks, sugar, chocolate and too much alcohol, which all act as stimulants and trigger blood sugar problems,

Increase your intake of fresh, locally grown and preferably organic fruits and vegetables.

Fermented soya-based foods are truly one of the best foods for managing the symptoms associated with the menopause. Soya contains isoflavones (phyto-estrogens), which have estrogen-like effects on the body and block the harmful effects of estrogens and xenoestrogens. There has been much misinformation written about soya, but soya foods in their traditional forms of miso, soya sauce and tempeh (a fermented form of soya) are all rich in isoflavones which have been proven to reduce the risk of developing cancers. But they are best eaten cooked.

Eat more organic tofu and use soya, rice or almond milks.

Isoflavones are also found in chickpeas, lentils, alfalfa, fennel, kidney beans, sunflower, pumpkin and sesame seeds, Brazil nuts, walnuts and linseeds. All seeds and their unrefined oils are rich in essential fatty adds which also help reduce joint pain, risk of heart disease.

Foods from the brassica vegetable family also help protect against estrogen-sensitive cancers, including breast cancer and cervix cancer, and balance hormones. These include cabbage, broccoli, pak choi. Brussels sprouts, cauliflower, kale, kohlrabi, mustard, rutabaga and turnips.

Brazil nuts and sesame seeds are a better source of calcium than cows' milk.

Live, low-fat yoghurt increases healthy bacteria in the gut, which aids absorption of nutrients from your diet.

Vitamin B12 has been shown to reduce irritability, bloating and headaches associated with the menopause and is found in oily fish, eggs and meats.

Potassium and pantothenic acid (vitamin B5) help support adrenal function. They are found in wholegrains such as brown rice, amaranth, barley, quinoa, salmon, tomatoes, broccoli, cauliflower, avocado, dried apricots, banana, cantaloupe melon, oranges and fish.

Use dried seaweeds such as kombu in your cooking and stir-fries, as seaweed is rich in iodine (which supports the thyroid) and calcium.

Eat organic foods including meat, chicken, vegetables and fruits to avoid ingesting too many toxins from herbicides and pesticides.

Folic acid found in wheatgerm, eggs, leafy greens, calves' and chicken liver, dried yeast and boiled beetroot is very important during the menopause to protect the bones.

Include garlic in your diet, which helps to keep cholesterol levels in check.

CBD oil works for menopause symptoms

CBD stands for cannabidiol oil. It is used to treat different symptoms even though its use is rather controversial. There is also some confusion as to how exactly the oil affects our bodies. The oil may have health benefits and such products that have the compound are legal in many places today.

What it is

CBD is a cannabinoid, a compound found in cannabis plant. The oil contains CBD concentrations and the uses vary greatly. In cannabis, the compound that is popular is delta 9 tetrahydrocannabinol or THC. It is an active ingredient found in marijuana. Marijuana has CBD and THCA and both have different effects.

THC alters the mind when one is smoking or cooking with it. This is because it is broken down by heat. Unlike THC, CBD isn't psychoactive. This means that your state of mind does not change with use. However, significant changes can be noted within the human body suggesting medical benefits.

Source

Hemp is a part of the cannabis plant and in most cases, it is not processed. This is where a lot of the CBD is extracted. Marijuana and hemp originate from cannabis sativa, but are quite different. Today, marijuana farmers are breeding plants so that they can have high THC levels. Hemp farmers do not need to modify plants and are used to create the CBD oil.

How it works

Cannabinoids affect the body by attaching themselves to different receptors. Some cannabinoids are produced by the body and there are the CB1 and CB2 receptors. CB1 receptors are located all through the body with a great number of them being in the brain. The receptors are responsible for mood, emotions, pain, movement, coordination, memories, appetite, thinking, and many other functions. THC affects these receptors.

As for the CB2 receptors, they are mainly in one's immune system and affect pain and inflammation. Even though CBD does not attach directly here, it directs the body to use cannabinoids more.

The benefits

CBD is beneficial to human health in different ways. It is a natural pain reliever and has anti-inflammatory properties. Over the counter drugs are used for pain relief and most people prefer a more natural alternative and this is where CBD oil comes in.

Research has shown that CBD provides a better treatment, especially for people with chronic pain.

There is also evidence that suggest that the use of CBD can be very helpful for anyone who is trying to quit smoking and dealing with drug withdrawals. In a study, it was seen that smokers who had inhalers that had CBD tended to smoke less than what was usual for them and without any further craving for cigarettes. CBD could be a great treatment for persons with addiction disorders especially to opioids.

There are many other medical conditions that are aided by CBD and they include epilepsy, LGA, Dravet syndrome, seizures and so on. More research is being conducted on the effects of CBD in the human body and the results are quite promising. The possibility of combating cancer and different anxiety disorders is also being looked at.

Natural Therapies For Menopause

Every woman will have to go through stages of her life where changes are inevitable. Probably one of the most unwanted stages is the menopausal stage. Not only does it sound fearful because of the accompanying discomfort of the symptoms but also because these symptoms are, especially when they are most unbearable, signs of a looming old age. The immense changes that happen physically can be very emotionally painful to some women. Who would celebrate the idea of physical symptoms that bring about hot flashes, mood swings, anxiety, feeling out of your primetime with the world or harboring the though that your reproductive years are over and very soon, you will feel weak, look old, and be the most unattractive woman.

Whether your menopause is a result of a reproductive illness or simply just part of the normal aging process, there is still hope that you can celebrate entering this stage of womanhood feeling and looking better because of reducing the symptoms. Estrogen replacement may be the solution but women can opt for natural remedies to alleviate the symptoms of menopause. Natural remedies for menopause include just the same basic things that we do to maintain good health. This includes lifestyle changes especially on the food we eat, exercise, and of course food and nutritional supplements or directly including in our diet herbs that are believed to be containing the same essential ingredients that hormonal replacement provides.

Before doing this though, it is always wise to consult a medical professional or your personal doctor regarding natural remedies for menopause. There might be some negative interaction with ongoing medication or just a simple allergy check on the food that are safe to eat. At the end of it, everything comes to its prime and if a woman has reached self actualization at the prime years of her life, there is no way that going through menopause should get in the way of aging gracefully and enjoying those golden years.

Over 300 different plants contain estrogenic substances. Although these are weak estrogens and are present only in tiny quantities, if foods containing them are consumed regularly, they can exert a mild estrogenic effect in humans.

Alfalfa contains a plant estrogen called coumestrol, which can actually cause infertility in animals that graze on large pastures of alfalfa grasses. Of all the plant estrogens, coumestrol is the most potent, although it is still 200 times weaker than human estrogens. The herb red clover also contains coumestrol and can be taken in the form of an herbal tea, or you can make fresh sprouts from red clover seeds. As some varieties of red clover are poisonous, however, it is best to obtain supplies from a reputable herbalist or health food store.

Soybeans, soybean sprouts, and flaxseed meal (crushed flaxseeds) are excellent sources of natural estrogens as well as of protein and essential fatty acids. They are definitely anti-aging foods for menopausal women. For a list of foods and herbs that are good sources of plant estrogens.

Menopausal Skin Care

Taking a proactive approach to menopausal skin care is the only way to maintain your skin's health during the years that hormonal changes wreck havoc with your body.

It's bad enough when your body becomes involuntarily possessed by an intermittent raging inferno but when you begin to notice the toll that menopause takes upon your skin then it is past time to take action! Serious action!

Post 40 something skin has a variety of needs, particularly as pre-menopausal symptoms begin.

This is the time to assess your skin care needs and proactively revise your daily skin care routine to include products that are specifically formulated for aging and menopausal skin concerns.

The simple secrets to maintaining healthy and youthful looking skin specifically includes:

- Stimulating the production of collagen

- Maintaining well hydrated skin

- Neutralizing free radical activity

- Encouraging the growth of new skin cells

- Utilizing products with effective clinically proven active anti-aging ingredients

There a variety of proven successful strategies that can be utilized to maximize the benefits of an effective facial rejuvenation regime for menopausal skin care needs.

It's bad enough that your body has betrayed you and turned into a perpetual raging volcano complete with a red hot flush that slowly flows up your body to explode out the top of your head. Not to mention the rivers of sweat that accompany a hot flash that drips and runs in an unappealing lava flow throughout the day and night or that your memory has gone on strike, the new crop of thick manly man's whiskers starting to sprout on the chin and upper lip, and that unexpected game of hide and seek that you have to play with your libido.

In particular, during the onset of menopause facial skin tends to become much dryer.

Of course that's not too surprising given the amount of sweating that occurs during those hot flashes and night sweats. As beautiful plump, taut skin gradually begins to lose its moisture content and elasticity the deterioration starts. Fine lines emerge that gradually deepen into wrinkles accentuated by cavernous sagging folds that demonstrate a disconcerting tendency to jiggle when you move. If all that isn't enough to contend with be forewarned, acne outbreaks can return with a vengeance!

Why does all this happen?

Throughout menopause a variety of hormonal changes occur; estrogen levels decrease, collagen cell production diminishes, blood circulation slows, moisture retention becomes less efficient and skin thickness actually begins to thin out.

Now that your body seems to have completely morphed into an entirely different creature by transforming itself into an unsightly limp, saggy, baggy version of your former self it is time to stage your revolt!

The first strategy is to make sure that you keep yourself well hydrated by drinking more water than you think is possible. Think of it like this, if you deprive a plant of sufficient water, what happens? The plant slowly begins to droop then starts to shrivel up into a dry, crinkled husk. Get the picture?

Menopausal skin needs moisture, lots of moisture, to keep it healthy.

Yes, it means making more frequent trips to the bathroom but it is well worth it in the long run. The rule of thumb is to drink enough liquid every day, (water is best), so that the urine is fairly clear. Seal in moisture after cleaning by using a rich moisturizer jammed packed with nutrients, antioxidants and facial rejuvenation ingredients, repeating applications throughout the day as needed. Misting the skin throughout the day will help keep it hydrated as well.

Next, refrain from using facial products that have detergent or astringents in them because that will contribute to drying out the skin. Switch to a cleanser and other skin care products that are rich in emollients and clinically proven active anti-aging ingredients. Use a toner to keep the skin clean as washing the face once a day is sufficient for most skin types.

Exfoliating becomes a key element of any facial rejuvenation regime in order to stimulate new skin cell renewal by exfoliating away the old dead cells that collect on the surface of the skin. Of course, it goes without saying that a critical component to menopausal skin care is sunscreen all year long. Protection against the UVA and

UVB rays of the sun is a must to prevent further skin damage as well as to diminish the destruction that free radical cause to the skin.

Finally, taking a holistic approach to skin care is truly the means to ensuring a youthful appearance as the years march along. Maintaining a healthful diet, exercising regularly, consuming alcohol in moderation, not smoking, and getting plenty of sleep will not only add years to your life but will improve your overall health and appearance.

The Best Strategy Of Alternative HRT, Exercise And Menopause Go Hand In Hand

Hormone replacement therapy or simply HRT is a process whereby a patient gets imbued with the hormones just in order to augment the lack of naturally occurring hormones. There are three major causes which makes a person to undergo HRT. These include HRT for menopause; HRT for gender-variant people and HRT for Hypogonadism.

In case of the HRT for the menopause it is designed for the women who are undergoing menopause. It is a known fact that menopause causes depression, mood swings, hot flashes, osteoporosis and can sometimes lead towards the fatal condition of dementia. In menopause there is a lessened secretion of progesterone and testosterone which not only diminishes libido but also a feeling of well-being amongst the women. Most commonly HRT is taken in the form of a pill. Various clinical experiments and longitudinal studies have suggested that an HRT can lessen the chances of fatal heart attack among the women.

Secondly, HRT is also suggested for those people who have difficulty in conforming to their natural sex. It is usually given during the childhood to ascertain the sex of the child or after sex change operation in the adults.

Finally when it comes to countering the side effects of Hypogonadism (usually among the males) this treatment is finally recommended. It is also recommended to the people who are diagnosed with some kind of testicular malfunctioning or testicular cancer or whose testis have undergone sever injury.

Like every other synthetic treatment the HRT also comes with certain risks. It has been found off late that long term use of HRT by women (for more than ten years) can lead towards an increased risk of heart attack. However here the risks are quite low and a low number of women, who have been undergoing HRT, may be at the risk of a Heart Attack. Moreover research also suggests that women who undergo HRT are under an increased risk of Ovarian Cancer as well. However, the ultimate decision about whether to go for HRT or not rests with the women in question. She must only proceed after a thorough deliberation about its side effects with the physician.

On the positive side, innumerable clinical findings suggest that women who undergo HRT greatly reduce the chance of osteoporosis as compared to those who do not.

In order to offset the side effects of HRT some doctors duly recommend the use of Low Dose Hormone Replacement therapy so that its side effects could be minimalized.

Yoga For Menopause Relief

Yoga exercise, an ancient process of healing, exerts a positive effect on well-being and health, simply by altering the way in which we think, feel as well as respond to daily life situations. Yoga is likewise an alternative cure for alleviating agony and stress. In fact, the workout is even tested to possess a relationship with the menstrual cycle of women. It's supposed to be excellent for Premenstrual Syndrome (PMS) as it is believed that the body needs a lot more stretching and breathing to have alleviation from the symptoms.

Menstruation, also referred to as the uterine cycle, is often a natural phenomenon in a woman's existence that takes place every 4 weeks from puberty to menopause. It is characterized by regular monthly vaginal discharge of blood together with cells coming from the uterine linings, discomfort, sleeping disorders, headache, becoming easily irritated, depression, or sometimes even chaotic behavior and suicidal tendencies. The menstrual cycle usually persists from 2 to 7 days. Girls go through hormonal adjustments during monthly period, and tend to become stressed during this period. Despite the fact that monthly period is normal, several women encounter a number of dilemmas during their monthly periods. Some experience Menstrual Cramps or Dysmenorrhea, or Premenstrual Syndrome.

A regular exercise of yoga ensures relief from pain, and steers the body and mind to the pink of well-being. A look into Hatha Yoga, which includes yoga poses, breathing, and meditation, extols its threefold blessing: health and fitness, well-being and long life. It is wise to draw from the effectiveness of yoga exercise, particularly for women during the phases of menstruation, menopause, pregnancy and pre-menstrual syndrome. In result, yoga helps to overcome the discomfort and pain involved during the vulnerable phases in a woman's life. It's appropriately stated, "Peace in the body gives poise in the mind".

Several yoga poses are revealed to relieve menstrual pain that could likewise support the body and mind adjust with stress, anxiety and depressive disorder causing you to feel peaceful and calm, and also empowering you to cope with psychological signs of PMS. A few asana or yoga poses that are determined helpful in dealing with monthly period disorders are: Kapalabhati, Sukhasana (Easy Pose), Bidalasana (Cat Pose), Dhanurasana (Bow Pose), Bhujangasana (Cobra Pose), Matsyasana (Fish Pose), Pavanamuktasana (Wind Relieving Pose), Anuloma Viloma (Alternate Nostril Breathing) and Shavasana or the Corpse Pose. The poses listed alleviate menstrual cramping, major bleeding, pelvic pain and the low back pain related to menses.

Thus, yoga exercise is certainly great for people affected by Premenstrual Syndrome (PMS) or going through monthly period. The postures and breathing exercises really can help to relax the mind, relax the body, extend the cramped muscle tissues, and also boost the mood. If combined with a healthy diet plan, then the entire body will get the energy needed to deal with the symptoms of PMS and cycles, making the combo among the cheapest and most trusted methods for treating menstrual dysfunctions compared to over the counter medication. However, a person must take care to go easy on the yoga exercise. Inversions and twists needs to be refrained from because these block the flow of the blood. The movement has to end completely before it's possible to resume the exercise of inversion. As soon as the flow ends, start with inversions. Also engaging in asanas that press the belly and physical exercise should be avoided.

Conclusion

All women at some point will go through the menopause and individual experiences will differ. The management of the menopause and its symptoms will depend on a number of factors including whether the menopause is natural or caused by surgery or another medical treatment; whether the menopause is early/premature; what symptoms appear and whether their severity impacts on quality of life and whether there are further risks such as osteoporosis as a result of the menopause.

Some women will choose a self-help 'natural' approach to symptom management while others will choose to go on HRT. For all women lifestyle factors such as diet, exercise, smoking and alcohol will play an important part in promoting general wellbeing and reducing the risks associated with the menopause.

Being informed from the start, seeking advice on options available and being supported and understood at work and at home should all help to ensure that this natural part of life passes as smoothly as possible with physical and mental good health being managed and sustained.

DISCLAIMER